FROM MANAGING TO CONQUERING EXOCRINE PANCREATIC INSUFFICIENCEY

Expert guide to Understanding EPI Causes, Decoding Symptoms, and Navigating Treatment Strategies for a Vibrant and Healthy Life

DR. DASHIELL DANIEL

The book "Exocrine Pancreatic Insufficiency" is an excellent resource for learning about the nuances of a disease that has a major impact on digestive health. This book is significant because it carefully examines exocrine pancreatic insufficiency (EPI) and offers a balanced viewpoint on the condition's definition and a critical understanding of its consequences. The introduction emphasizes how important it is to understand the nuances of EPI, laying the groundwork for a detailed investigation.

The first chapter explores the architecture and physiology of the pancreas, explaining the anatomical details and intricate functions of this essential organ. The book provides a fundamental understanding of pancreatic function by delving deeply into the role of enzymes in digestion, which paves the way for further chapters.

The discourse is further elevated in Chapter 2, which delves into the fundamentals of EPI, including its description, causes, and a detailed investigation of its pathophysiology. This section plays a crucial role in deciphering the typical symptoms and indicators linked to EPI, promoting a sophisticated understanding of the illness.

Chapter 3 then proceeds to traverse the terrain of diagnosis, explaining the different modalities—such as imaging examinations, laboratory testing, and clinical evaluation—that are necessary for precisely identifying EPI. The reader's comprehension is further enhanced by Chapters 4 and 5, which break down the fundamental reasons for EPI and outline a variety of treatment alternatives, such as enzyme replacement therapy and dietary changes.

In Chapter 6, the emphasis is shifted to the practical aspects of living with eating disorders (EPI). The chapter provides information on coping techniques for food limitations, supportive therapies, and lifestyle adaptations. The following chapters explore the possible side effects and prognosis of end-stage renal illness (EPI), offering a comprehensive picture of the difficulties patients may encounter and long-term care options.

The final chapter delves into the ever-changing field of EPI research and development, providing insights into current projects, new treatments, and technological developments. By showcasing the ongoing advancements in the area and opening the door for upcoming developments in the treatment of exocrine pancreatic insufficiency, this section acts as a ray of hope.

All things considered, "Exocrine Pancreatic Insufficiency" is regarded as a landmark work that not only spreads important information regarding EPI but also fills the knowledge gap between theory and actual management. It is a priceless tool for researchers, medical experts, and anyone looking to gain a deeper comprehension of this intricate gastrointestinal ailment.

Overview

A complicated medical illness known as exocrine pancreatic insufficiency (EPI) is defined by the pancreas secreting insufficient amounts of digestive enzymes, which impairs nutrition absorption and digestion. Enzymes that are vital for the digestion of proteins, lipids, and carbohydrates include lipase, amylase, and protease, all of which are produced by the pancreas. EPI develops when this exocrine function is hampered, leading to a series of gastrointestinal issues. Healthcare workers must grasp the complexities of EPI to diagnose patients more quickly, manage them more effectively, and provide better treatment for them.

Exocrine Pancreatic Insufficiency (Epi) Definition

Exocrine pancreatic insufficiency is characterized by the pancreas's inadequate synthesis and release of digestive enzymes, which impairs food absorption and digestion. The primary impact of this deficit is on the breakdown of macronutrients, which results in malabsorption of carbs, proteins, and fats. Pancreatic tumors, cystic fibrosis, chronic pancreatitis, and other disorders that impair pancreatic function can all be underlying causes of EPI. Reduced enzyme activity affects digestion, leading to symptoms like diarrhea, weight loss, and deficits in certain nutrients.

The Value Of Comprehending EPI

In the field of medicine, understanding exocrine pancreatic insufficiency is essential for several reasons. First off, because EPI's symptoms are vague and can be mistaken for other gastrointestinal conditions, it is frequently misdiagnosed. Enhanced consciousness among medical practitioners is essential for timely and precise diagnosis, avoiding postponements at the start of therapy. Understanding the significance of EPI also helps to explain how it affects patients' general health, nutritional condition, and quality of life.

Additionally, in the setting of related disorders, EPI identification is crucial. For example, EPI is often associated with chronic pancreatitis, a disease in which the pancreas becomes inflamed. Comprehending this relationship is essential for an all-encompassing patient care strategy since treating the underlying ailment becomes critical to reducing EPI symptoms. Furthermore, a focused therapy approach that addresses the underlying illness, as well as any downstream problems, is made possible by the identification of EPI in conditions like cystic fibrosis.

EPI's Pathophysiology

The pathophysiology of exocrine pancreatic insufficiency is centered on the disturbance of pancreatic enzyme secretion, which in turn leads to a reduction in the ability to properly digest nutrients. Under normal physiological conditions, the pancreas produces dormant digestive enzymes that are subsequently activated in the duodenum. This process is hampered in EPI by conditions such as pancreatic injury, ductal blockage, or genetic abnormalities that alter the synthesis of enzymes. As a result, malabsorption and diarrhea are caused by the transit of undigested food into the colon due to insufficient digestion of macronutrients in the small intestine.

Chronic inflammation, as in chronic pancreatitis, or other disorders affecting the pancreatic tissue frequently causes the pancreatic damage that underlies EPI. Fibrosis and scarring brought on by inflammation might hinder the pancreas' natural architecture and further jeopardize its exocrine function. Comprehending the pathophysiological mechanisms causing enzyme secretion deficiencies (EPI) is essential for customizing therapy strategies, focusing on individual flaws, and addressing the underlying causes.

Presentation Of Clinical Data And Diagnosis

Exocrine pancreatic insufficiency can manifest clinically in a variety of ways, which makes diagnosis difficult. Abdominal pain, bloating, steatorrhea, weight loss, and nutritional deficits are typical symptoms.

However, because these symptoms might be confused with those of other gastrointestinal conditions, a thorough diagnosis process is required. To reach a conclusive diagnosis, medical practitioners need to take into account the patient's history, do a comprehensive physical examination, and combine laboratory and imaging findings.

Fecal elastase is frequently used in laboratory testing to quantify the amount of elastase in the stool, which serves as an indirect indicator of pancreatic enzyme activity. Blood testing can also show dietary inadequacies, like low fat-soluble vitamin levels. Imaging tests that can detect structural anomalies in the pancreas include computed tomography (CT) scans and abdominal ultrasonography.

For a more thorough assessment of the pancreatic ducts, endoscopic techniques like magnetic resonance cholangiopancreatography (MRCP) or endoscopic retrograde cholangiopancreatography (ERCP) may be used.

Strategies For EPI Treatment

A multimodal strategy is used to treat exocrine pancreatic insufficiency with the goals of correcting dietary inadequacies, symptom relief, and underlying cause identification.

The mainstay of care involves using oral enzyme supplements to replenish pancreatic enzymes. These supplements help with the digestion of fats, carbohydrates, and proteins because they contain the enzymes lipase, amylase, and protease, respectively.

Enzyme replacement must be timed and dosed correctly to maximize its effectiveness.

Dietary changes are essential for controlling Epstein-Barr syndrome (EPI), with a focus on a diet that is readily digested and well-balanced. Patients are frequently told to eat less fat in their diet and to think about taking supplements of fat-soluble vitamins.

It is imperative to oversee and address dietary deficits to avert protracted issues linked to malabsorption.

When EPI results from an underlying illness, such as cystic fibrosis or chronic pancreatitis, treating the underlying disease is essential to managing the condition well. This can entail ductal blockage relief procedures, anti-inflammatory drugs, or pain management. A complete and patient-centered strategy requires collaboration with experts in nutrition, gastroenterology, and other pertinent domains.

The diagnosis and management of exocrine pancreatic insufficiency provide considerable problems because of the wide range of clinical presentations and underlying causes.

Healthcare practitioners must have a solid understanding of EPI to overcome these obstacles and develop efficient treatment plans and timely, accurate diagnoses.

Novel insights and therapeutic methods for persons affected by EPI may be provided by breakthroughs in the field as research into the complexity of pancreas function and its involvement in digestive health continues.

CHAPTER ONE

PANCREAS' ANATOMY AND PHYSIOLOGY

As both an endocrine and an exocrine gland, the pancreas is an essential organ in the human body that helps to maintain homeostasis. The pancreas has a complex structure made up of both endocrine and exocrine components. The majority of the pancreas, known as the exocrine component, is in charge of creating digestive enzymes.

The endocrine portion, which is represented by the islets of Langerhans, secretes hormones like glucagon and insulin. This dual role emphasizes how important the pancreas is for controlling metabolism.

Acinar cells, which secrete digestive enzymes, and ducts, which carry these enzymes to the duodenum, make up the structural organization of the exocrine pancreas. Amylases, lipases, and proteases are among the inactive enzyme precursors called zymogens that are released into the pancreatic ducts by the acinar cells. Following their activation in the duodenum, these zymogens aid in the digesting process by breaking down proteins, lipids, and carbs. For the best possible digestion processes, the precise coordination of enzyme release is made possible by the complex structure of the pancreas.

In terms of function, the pancreas is involved in both digestion and the absorption of nutrients.

The exocrine pancreas secretes digestive enzymes that are vital for dissolving complicated foods into more palatable parts. Amylases help break down proteins, lipases help break down fats, and amylases help break down carbohydrates. For the body to absorb and use nutrients for energy, growth, and maintenance, the pancreas helps to convert food that is swallowed.

The pancreas is a key producer of these catalytic agents, which are essential for digestion. Pancreatic amylase is one of the amylases that breaks down glucose and starch into simpler sugars like maltose.

Triglycerides are the target of lipases like pancreatic lipase, which breaks them down into fatty acids and glycerol.

Trypsin and chymotrypsin are examples of proteases that target proteins and break them down into amino acids. This well-coordinated enzymatic action guarantees effective digestion, allowing the body to absorb vital nutrients from food.

When the pancreas is unable to create enough digestive enzymes, it can lead to exocrine pancreatic insufficiency (EPI), which can impair the body's ability to absorb nutrients. Numerous conditions, such as cystic fibrosis, pancreatic cancer, or chronic pancreatitis, can produce this shortage. The health of an individual is significantly impacted by the structural and functional abnormalities linked to EPI.

Inflammation or injury to the pancreas may jeopardize its structural integrity in situations of EPI. Acinar cells and ducts may be affected by fibrotic alterations in the pancreatic tissue as a result of chronic pancreatitis, a condition marked by ongoing inflammation.

This structural change impairs the pancreas's capacity to generate and distribute enzymes efficiently, which adds to the deficiency seen in EPI.

The insufficient release of digestive enzymes, which interferes with the regular digestive process, is the functional element of EPI.

When necessary nutrients like proteins, lipids, and carbs are not adequately absorbed and broken down in the small intestine, it results in malabsorption.

As a result, symptoms including diarrhea, weight loss, and vitamin shortages may be present in people with EPI, which is indicative of the body's poor use of ingested nutrients.

Enzymes play a critical part in digestion, and a lack of them in the EPI can have a domino impact on health. Insufficient amylase activity causes a condition known as carbohydrate malabsorption, which allows undigested carbohydrates to enter the colon. Here, the carbohydrates work as substrates for the fermentation of bacteria, which results in the generation of gasses and osmotically active chemicals that aggravate diarrhea and cause discomfort in the abdomen.

Furthermore, malabsorption of dietary lipids occurs as a result of poor fat digestion in EPI. Steatorrhea, a defining symptom of EPI, results from the excretion of undigested fats in the stool as a result of this. Steatorrhea can lead to nutritional deficits due to improper absorption of fat-soluble vitamins (A, D, E, and K), which are sometimes accompanied by foul-smelling, oily feces.

Because there is insufficient protease activity in EPI, protein malabsorption occurs, allowing undigested proteins to enter the colon. These proteins are broken down by bacteria in the colon, which results in compounds that increase the osmotic load and worsen diarrhea.

The overall effect of EPI on the malabsorption of nutrients highlights the role of the pancreas in preserving the body's nutritional state and general health.

In summary, the pancreas's exocrine function—where the synthesis of digestive enzymes is essential for the breakdown and absorption of nutrients—is closely related to both its structure and physiology. Malabsorption of proteins, lipids, and carbohydrates results from this mechanism being disrupted in exocrine pancreatic insufficiency (EPI), which has serious health effects. Gaining knowledge about the anatomical and functional features of the pancreas improves our understanding of EPI and facilitates the creation of focused therapies aimed at reducing its effects on the absorption of nutrients and general health.

CHAPTER TWO
UNDERSTANDING EXOGENOUS PANCREATIC INSUFFICIENCY

The disorder known as exocrine pancreatic insufficiency (EPI) is defined by the pancreas secreting insufficient amounts of digestive enzymes, which impairs digestion and the absorption of nutrients. Enzymes that are vital for the digestion of fats, carbohydrates, and proteins include lipase, amylase, and protease, all of which are produced primarily by the pancreas.

EPI is caused by an impaired pancreatic exocrine function, which impacts nutrition absorption and the digestive process as a whole.

Meaning And Origins Of EPI

The pancreas produces insufficient amounts of digestive enzymes, which is known as exocrine pancreatic insufficiency.

Gastrointestinal problems, various systemic ailments, and pancreatic diseases can be classified as the chief causes of EPI. One of the main causes of EPI is chronic pancreatitis, a disorder characterized by pancreatic inflammation. EPI can also result from a hereditary illness called cystic fibrosis, which affects the pancreas among other organs. Pancreatic cancer, autoimmune disorders that impact the pancreas, and specific surgical procedures that may impair pancreatic function are additional possible reasons.

EPI's Pathophysiology

The pathogenesis of exocrine pancreatic insufficiency is centered on the impairment of the secretion of pancreatic enzymes and the subsequent processes involved in digestion. Prolonged inflammation affects pancreatic tissue in diseases such as chronic pancreatitis, impairing the production and secretion of digesting enzymes. Exocrine function is further compromised by this injury, which results in the replacement of functional tissue with fibrous tissue.

A genetic mutation that causes cystic fibrosis alters the synthesis of a protein that is involved in the movement of chloride ions, thickening secretions in the pancreas among other organs. The pancreatic ducts are blocked by this thickness, which prevents enzymes from entering the digestive system. As a result, malabsorption and nutritional deficits are brought on by the partial digestion of nutrients.

Typical Signs And Symptoms

Exocrine pancreatic insufficiency can present with a variety of symptoms, many of which are gastrointestinal and systemic in nature. The symptoms of the digestive system include bloating, flatulence, diarrhea, steatorrhea (fatty stools), and stomach pain. Its distinctive look is caused by the emission of undigested fat in the stool, which results from insufficient fat digestion.

EPI frequently results in weight loss because the body is unable to absorb vital nutrients.

Moreover, dietary deficits, such as those in fat-soluble vitamins (A, D, E, and K), may be experienced by people with EPI. Beyond the gastrointestinal tract, systemic symptoms can impact general health and well-being. Due to the body's incapacity to absorb essential nutrients, these could include weakening in the muscles, weariness, and an overall feeling of malaise.

Identification And Handling

A combination of imaging techniques, laboratory testing, and clinical assessment is used to diagnose exocrine pancreatic insufficiency. Pancreatic enzyme levels in the stool can be measured by stool tests, like the fecal elastase test, which yields important diagnostic data. Imaging methods such as magnetic resonance imaging (MRI) and computed tomography (CT) scans can identify structural anomalies in the pancreas. Blood tests can evaluate associated abnormalities and inadequacies in nutrition.

Following a diagnosis, the goals of EPI care are to treat the underlying cause, reduce symptoms, and guarantee adequate nutrient absorption. The mainstay of EPI management is enzyme replacement therapy, which involves taking supplements of pancreatic enzymes with meals to help with digestion.

Dietary changes could also be advised to maximize nutritional intake and lessen symptoms. When EPI results from an underlying ailment, like chronic pancreatitis, treating the underlying disease becomes essential to the overall therapy strategy.

The complicated disorder known as exocrine pancreatic insufficiency has a variety of etiologist and profound effects on nutrition intake and digestion.

It is essential to comprehend the pathophysiology, definition, causes, and typical symptoms of EPI to make an accurate diagnosis and provide appropriate treatment.

There is hope for better results for those impacted by pancreatic dysfunction as a study into the condition's complexities continues and new developments in diagnostic techniques and treatment approaches are made possible.

CHAPTER THREE
EXOCRINE PANCREATIC INSUFFICIENCY DIAGNOSIS

The diagnosis of exocrine pancreatic insufficiency (EPI) is difficult because of the disorder's numerous, frequently subtle clinical symptoms. Diagnosis is a multidisciplinary process that includes imaging scans, laboratory testing, and clinical assessment.

Clinical Evaluation: An essential part of diagnosing exocrine pancreatic insufficiency is clinical assessment. Patients may arrive with vague symptoms including diarrhea, bloating, and stomach pain. It is essential to get a thorough medical history that addresses alcohol intake, food habits, and any prior pancreatic conditions. Because digestive symptoms might mimic those of other ailments, a thorough examination is necessary to distinguish EPI from conditions such as irritable bowel syndrome.

Weight loss and nutritional inadequacies are examples of related symptoms that doctors should take into account as they might offer important hints.

A physical examination may identify symptoms such as steatorrhea, nutritional deficits, or pain in the abdomen that are suggestive of malabsorption. It is crucial to remember that a multifaceted approach is required for a definitive diagnosis, as clinical evaluation alone may not be sufficient in this regard.

Laboratory Tests: An essential part of the exocrine pancreatic insufficiency diagnostic strategy is the laboratory test. One stool-based test that stands out as a trustworthy and non-invasive marker for EPI is fecal elastase-1. The pancreatic elastase enzyme, which is stable throughout the gastrointestinal tract, is measured by this test.

The diagnosis of EPI is confirmed by a low fecal elastase-1 level, which denotes insufficient pancreatic enzyme activity.

Serum trypsinogen and chymotrypsin levels are two further laboratory tests. However, these tests don't have the same sensitivity and specificity as fecal elastase-1. Additionally, blood tests can be used to evaluate nutritional deficiencies brought on by malabsorption, such as low levels of minerals and fat-soluble vitamins (A, D, E, and K).

Understanding that no one test is infallible and that laboratory results must be evaluated in conjunction with clinical findings is crucial.

 To improve diagnostic accuracy, more testing could be necessary in situations when the diagnosis is still unclear.

Imaging Studies: By helping to visualize the pancreatic anatomy and identify structural anomalies, imaging studies play a crucial role in the diagnosis of exocrine pancreatic insufficiency. Initial imaging using abdominal ultrasonography is a frequently used technique. It offers a non-invasive evaluation of the pancreas, identifying alterations in its size, form, or existence of pancreatic cysts.

Ultrasonography is frequently used in conjunction with other imaging modalities since it may not have the sensitivity needed to identify mild cases of EPI.

A more thorough assessment of the pancreas is provided by computed tomography (CT) scans, which aid in the detection of calcifications or pancreatic atrophy. Another useful technique that produces high-resolution images without subjecting the patient to ionizing radiation is magnetic resonance imaging (MRI).

These imaging tests help rule out other possible causes of pancreatic dysfunction and add to the overall evaluation of pancreatic anatomy.

When it comes to seeing the pancreatic ductal system, endoscopic retrograde cholangiopancreatography (ERCP) is still considered the gold standard. Despite being invasive, it makes the pancreatic and ductal structures directly visible, making it easier to find strictures or other obstructions that may be causing EPI.

A synergistic strategy that includes imaging scans, laboratory testing, and clinical evaluation is used to diagnose exocrine pancreatic insufficiency. For a thorough understanding of the patient's state, careful integration of different modalities is necessary, guaranteeing an accurate diagnosis and prompt implementation of suitable management methods.

SECTION FOUR
FUNDAMENTAL REASONS FOR EXOGENOUS PANTREAMIC INSUFFICIENCY

The disorder known as exocrine pancreatic insufficiency (EPI) is typified by insufficient pancreatic enzyme production and secretion, which is necessary for the breakdown of proteins, lipids, and carbohydrates. A variety of symptoms, including weight loss, steatorrhea, and nutritional deficiencies, are brought on by the impairment of these digestive enzymes, which causes malabsorption and nutritional deficiencies.

This thorough investigation will look at pancreatic cancer, cystic fibrosis, chronic pancreatitis, and other contributing variables as it delves into the fundamental origins of EPI.

Chronic pancreatitis is a chronic inflammatory condition of the pancreas marked by irreparable damage to pancreatic tissue, fibrosis, and continuous inflammation. It is a key contributor to exocrine pancreatic insufficiency. The long-term inflammatory process causes scar tissue to replace functioning pancreatic tissue, impairing the organ's capacity to appropriately generate and release digestion enzymes. When the pancreas sustains severe damage, leading to insufficient release of enzymes including amylase, lipase, and protease, EPI frequently develops in the final stages of chronic pancreatitis. The clinical signs of EPI are caused by the pancreas's inability to function normally due to an inflammatory cascade and fibrotic alterations.

An autosomal recessive hereditary disease primarily affecting the digestive and respiratory systems is called cystic fibrosis (CF). Mutations in the CFTR gene cause the illness, which is characterized by the development of thick, sticky mucus that clogs several ducts and passages, including the pancreatic ducts. Mucus buildup in the pancreatic ducts inhibits the regular flow of pancreatic enzymes into the duodenum.

As a result, people with cystic fibrosis frequently experience difficulties digesting and absorbing nutrients from their diet due to exocrine pancreatic insufficiency. The genetic basis of EPI and the complex interaction between genetic variables and pancreatic function are highlighted by the link found between mutations in the CFTR gene and EPI.

Exocrine pancreatic insufficiency can also arise as a result of pancreatic cancer, a deadly disease with high morbidity and mortality. The pancreatic ducts may become blocked by a cancerous tumor in the pancreas, preventing the intestines from receiving adequate amounts of digestion enzymes. Furthermore, healthy pancreatic tissue may be invaded and destroyed by pancreatic cancer, severely impairing the organ's capacity to produce and secrete digestive enzymes. Tumors that obstruct the pancreatic ducts are more likely to develop endoplasmic prion illness (EPI), and the location and size of the tumor are important factors in determining the effect on pancreatic function.

Diabetes mellitus, pancreatic surgery, and some drugs are other causes that can lead to exocrine pancreatic insufficiency. Diabetes mellitus—more specifically, type 3c diabetes—is linked to pancreatic damage as a result of persistent inflammation, which compromises exocrine function.

The ability of the pancreas to produce digestive enzymes may be diminished by pancreatic procedures, such as pancreatectomy or surgery for pancreatic injuries, which can cause the loss of functional pancreatic tissue.

Certain pharmaceuticals have been linked to EPI by influencing pancreatic enzyme secretion or preventing the release of cholecystokinin, a hormone that promotes the production of pancreatic enzymes.

Examples of these medications include some antiepileptic drugs and long-term usage of proton pump inhibitors.

To sum up, exocrine pancreatic insufficiency is a complex illness with a range of underlying causes. The development of pancreatic function and many etiological factors are intricately linked, as seen by the important contributions of chronic pancreatitis, cystic fibrosis, pancreatic cancer, and other factors. Comprehending these fundamental reasons is essential for precise identification, efficient handling, and enhanced results for those impacted by exocrine pancreatic insufficiency.

CHAPTER FIVE

TREATMENT OPTIONS FOR EXOGENOUS PANCREATIC INSUFFICIENCY

The disorder known as exocrine pancreatic insufficiency (EPI) is defined by the pancreas producing insufficient amounts of digestive enzymes, which impairs digestion and the absorption of nutrients. A multimodal strategy involving dietary adjustments, enzyme replacement therapy (ERT), and addressing underlying causes is necessary for the effective management of epilepsy.

One of the most important treatments for exocrine pancreatic insufficiency is enzyme replacement therapy or ERT. The main goal of ERT is to replenish the lacking digestive enzymes, like protease, amylase, and lipase, which are necessary for the breakdown of proteins, lipids, and carbohydrates, respectively.

For this reason, pancreatic enzyme supplements, or PES, are frequently administered.

These supplements, which come in capsule form most of the time, are made of concentrated enzymes that come from other or porcine sources. Because lipase is a crucial component in the malabsorption of fats, its lack is particularly significant. It is recommended that patients take these supplements with meals to support healthy digestion and absorption of nutrients.

Essential components of ERT management include tracking treatment response, modifying enzyme dosage according to patient requirements, and controlling any possible side effects.

Dietary changes are essential for the treatment of exocrine pancreatic insufficiency. Dietary changes can help EPI patients feel better nutritionally and reduce symptoms, as they frequently have trouble digesting specific nutrients. Because EPI has decreased fat digestion, dietary fat intake may need to be restricted.

Additionally, eating a diet high in proteins and carbs that are quickly digested may be advantageous.

To facilitate digestion, patients are advised to eat smaller, more frequent meals. Healthcare providers may also advise against consuming particular foods, such as fatty or high-fat foods, as they are known to be more difficult to digest.

Based on each patient's unique nutritional requirements and the severity of their EPI, dietary recommendations should be customized.

A further crucial component of treating EPI is managing its underlying causes. Comprehensive management of pancreatic insufficiency requires the identification and treatment of its underlying cause. EPI can be exacerbated by long-term illnesses like pancreatic cancer, cystic fibrosis, and chronic pancreatitis. There are several different approaches to treating underlying problems, such as lifestyle changes, medication treatments, or surgical operations. To treat blockage or structural problems, for example, controlling chronic pancreatitis may entail lifestyle modifications, pain management, and in certain circumstances, surgery. Enzyme supplements, respiratory care, and nutritional support are all important components of a comprehensive treatment plan for cystic fibrosis, a hereditary illness that affects numerous organ systems. Surgery, chemotherapy, and radiation therapy may be used in combination when pancreatic cancer is the underlying cause of the condition.

In summary, treating exocrine pancreatic insufficiency necessitates a multifaceted strategy that takes into account both the condition's underlying causes and symptoms. To compensate for insufficient digestive enzymes, enzyme replacement treatment is essential. To maximize effectiveness, dosage modifications and close monitoring are required. Dietary changes are essential for enhancing nutrient intake and facilitating digestion. An individualized strategy that may involve medication, lifestyle changes, or surgery is required to manage underlying causes, such as cystic fibrosis or chronic pancreatitis.

To provide the best possible management of exocrine pancreatic insufficiency, customize treatment plans to each patient's needs, and enhance the overall quality of life, healthcare professionals and patients must work together.

CHAPTER SIX
LIVING WITH EXOGENOUS PANCREATIC INSUFFICIENCY

There are many obstacles that people with exocrine pancreatic insufficiency (EPI) have to deal with daily. This disorder has a major effect on nutrition absorption and digestion because of insufficient pancreatic synthesis and secretion of digestive enzymes. Making lifestyle changes that improve overall well-being becomes essential as people deal with the effects of EPI.

6.1 Lifestyle Modifications: To reduce symptoms and improve health outcomes, managing end-stage renal illness (EPI) requires significant lifestyle changes. To ease the strain on the weakened digestive system, patients are frequently instructed to follow a planned diet that involves frequent, smaller meals. It's also critical to stay away from foods that are high in fat and difficult to digest because they can make symptoms worse.

It is recommended to engage in regular physical activity to support gastrointestinal motility and help maintain a healthy body weight.

Avoiding excessive alcohol usage is also crucial because alcohol can exacerbate pancreatic dysfunction. Essentially, the key to effectively addressing the issues presented by EPI is adopting a comprehensive lifestyle that includes dietary modifications and activity levels.

6.2 Dealing with Dietary Restrictions: Given the pancreas's reduced capacity to create digestive enzymes, careful attention to dietary practices is the cornerstone of managing epilepsy.

Pancreatic enzyme replacement treatment (PERT), which involves supplementing patients with enzymes like lipase, protease, and amylase before meals, is frequently administered to patients. This makes up for the inadequacies in endogenous enzyme production by aiding in the digestion of proteins, lipids, and carbs.

The PERT regimen must be understood and followed to maximize nutrient absorption and prevent malnutrition. Furthermore, it could be necessary for people with EPI to keep a food journal to track how they react to certain foods and pinpoint triggers that make their symptoms worse. Despite the difficulties brought on by EPI, this self-awareness is essential for adjusting the diet to each person's demands and guaranteeing a sufficient intake of nutrients.

6.3 Supportive Therapies: In addition to dietary and lifestyle changes, supportive therapies are essential for improving the quality of life for people with EPI. Since the illness is persistent, psychological support is essential because it can cause anxiety and emotional anguish.

Patients can exchange experiences, coping mechanisms, and insights in counseling and support groups, which promotes a feeling of belonging and understanding. Additionally, healthcare professionals are essential in informing patients about the ailment, its consequences, and the significance of following treatment plans. Scheduling routine follow-up appointments allows for the monitoring of treatment efficacy and necessary modifications to the management plan. To further ensure that people with EPI obtain enough macro- and micronutrients and avoid malnutrition and its consequences, nutritional counseling is frequently included.

All things considered, a comprehensive strategy for supporting therapies includes not only the physiological aspects of managing electroencephalograms (EPIs) but also the psychological and educational elements that are part of a patient-centered, holistic care paradigm.

To sum up, managing dietary limitations, adopting supportive therapies, and changing one's lifestyle are all necessary aspects of living with exocrine pancreatic insufficiency. To effectively manage the problems offered by EPI and maximize their overall well-being, people must integrate these notions.

People with EPI can manage the intricacies of their condition and lead satisfying lives with the help of a supportive healthcare environment, individualized dietary modifications, and adherence to recommended medicines.

CHAPTER SEVEN
INTRICACIES AND EXTENDED PROSPECTS

The disorder known as exocrine pancreatic insufficiency (EPI) is defined by the pancreas producing insufficient amounts of digestive enzymes, which compromises digestion and nutrient absorption. It is essential to comprehend the complex nature of EPI as we delve into its complexities.

There are many different potential EPI consequences, all of which have the potential to seriously harm a person's health and general well-being. Malnutrition is a prominent outcome that arises from the compromised absorption of vital nutrients, including proteins, lipids, and fat-soluble vitamins. This malabsorption can cause nutritional shortages, weight loss, and muscle wastage, which can lead to a host of other health problems.

Furthermore, the patient may become deficient in vitamins A, D, E, and K as a result of the unabsorbed nutrients, which would increase their susceptibility to infections, bone diseases, and irregular blood coagulation.

Moreover, gastrointestinal issues may arise because of the chronic nature of EPI. Steatorrhea is a frequent symptom that is defined by an abundance of fat in the feces.

This results in diarrhea, stomach discomfort, and gas in addition to causing malabsorption of nutrients. Secondary disorders like pancreatitis and pancreatic fibrosis may arise as a result of the ongoing inflammation brought on by the weakened digestive system.

The prognosis for people with EPI may worsen as a result of these problems, requiring extensive care techniques.

For those with an extended period of illness (EPI), managing the related complications and treating the underlying causes will require a multifaceted strategy. For those who are impacted, the prognosis and long-term care are crucial factors in determining their quality of life. Enzyme replacement treatment (ERT), which seeks to supplement the lacking digestive enzymes and facilitate adequate digestion and food absorption, is a proactive approach to managing extrapyramidal syndrome (EPI). But problems might also occur, like varying responses to ERT, changing dosages, and other adverse effects, which calls for a cautious and individualized approach to therapy.

Furthermore, the foundation of long-term care is dietary interventions. A well-balanced, nutrient-dense diet with an emphasis on readily digested meals is frequently recommended to patients.

The objectives of this dietary adjustment are to improve nutritional status, lessen gastrointestinal discomfort, and lessen the effects of malabsorption. To customize dietary advice to each patient's specific needs, healthcare professionals—dietitians and gastroenterologists, in particular—must work together.

It's important to consider the psychological effects of EPI in addition to its physical components.

The chronic nature of the illness and the symptoms it causes can have a serious negative effect on a patient's general well-being and mental health. Alongside the physical symptoms of EPI, there may be accompanying feelings of anxiety, despair, and decreased well-being.

To empower people to manage the illness over time, a comprehensive strategy should include psychological assistance, therapy, and education.

Sustained observation and investigation are essential elements of long-term EPI management. This entails evaluating the patient's reaction to the treatment, modifying the therapeutic approach as necessary, and taking care of any new issues that may arise. Therapeutic decisions are guided by routine laboratory testing, imaging scans, and clinical evaluations, which help follow the condition's course.

For people living with EPI, thorough care and the best possible long-term results depend on the cooperative efforts of a multidisciplinary healthcare team.

To sum up, exocrine pancreatic insufficiency poses a challenging clinical situation with far-reaching consequences for those who are impacted. Beyond the digestive tract, nutritional condition, general health, and psychological well-being are among the possible side effects of EPI.

The prognosis and long-term management approaches play a critical role in reducing these problems and improving the quality of life for people with end-stage kidney illness.

Optimizing outcomes and addressing the various obstacles this condition presents require a thorough, multifaceted approach that incorporates medical, dietary, and psychological interventions.

CHAPTER 8
RESEARCH AND DEVELOPMENTS IN ETHANOL PRODUCTION

The disorder known as exocrine pancreatic insufficiency (EPI) is characterized by insufficient pancreatic enzyme secretion or synthesis, which impairs nutritional absorption and digestion. Several gastrointestinal symptoms, such as diarrhea, bloating, abdominal pain, and malnutrition, can result from this condition. Understanding the biology of EPI and creating efficient diagnostic and treatment strategies have advanced significantly in recent years.

Research Still Ahead: The goal of the current investigation into exocrine pancreatic insufficiency is to learn more about the cellular and molecular processes that underlie the illness.

The goal of research is to pinpoint the precise genetic, environmental, and immunological elements that contribute to the onset of EPI.

Researchers are looking into how pancreatic ductal and acinar cells secrete enzymes and how malfunction in these cells can result in insufficient synthesis of enzymes. Another area of ongoing research is to improve early diagnosis and track the progression of disease by identifying novel biomarkers.

In addition, studies are looking into the interactions between inflammatory bowel disease, cystic fibrosis, and chronic pancreatitis, among other gastrointestinal conditions. Gaining knowledge of the intricate relationships between various disorders could help develop focused treatment plans. The involvement of the gut microbiome in EPI is also gaining attention since changes in the microbial composition may affect pancreas function and worsen symptoms.

Emerging Therapies and Technology: With the advent of cutting-edge therapies and technology, the landscape of treatment for exocrine pancreatic insufficiency has changed. While pancreatic enzyme replacement therapy (PERT) is still the mainstay for treating end-stage pancreatitis (EPI), researchers are working hard to create patient-friendly and more potent formulations. The goal of developments in enzyme encapsulation technologies is to increase the bioavailability and stability of enzymes for the best possible gastrointestinal tract absorption and digestion.

Beyond conventional PERT, pharmaceutical strategies that focus on certain pathways related to the secretion and control of enzymes are gaining popularity. The potential of small chemical activators and inhibitors to alter pancreatic function and treat the underlying causes of EPI is being studied. Certain inherited forms of EPI may be cured using gene therapy, which can address genetic defects linked to the disorder.

Technological developments in diagnostic techniques, in addition to treatment approaches, are improving our capacity to identify and track EPI.

For evaluating pancreatic morphology and function, non-invasive imaging methods like magnetic resonance imaging (MRI) and elastography are being investigated. Accurate and prompt EPI diagnosis is facilitated by the development of more sensitive and specific biomarker testing, such as pancreatic imaging methods and fecal elastase.

CONCLUSION

In conclusion, there is a dynamic and changing landscape in the understanding and treatment of exocrine pancreatic insufficiency, which is reflected in the current research and developing therapeutics. The investigation of the immunological, molecular, and genetic components of EPI lays the groundwork for personalized medicine strategies that customize treatments to the unique underlying reasons in each patient.

Improvements in patient outcomes and medication adherence are demonstrated by the introduction of innovative formulations and breakthroughs in pancreatic enzyme replacement therapy. The use of cutting-edge diagnostic techniques supports early and accurate EPI diagnosis, facilitating prompt action and averting long-term problems, as technology continues to play a critical role in healthcare.

Even if there are still obstacles to overcome, such as the requirement for longer-term outcome evaluations and more thorough clinical studies, the advancements in EPI research provide affected people hope for a better quality of life. Future therapeutic approaches are expected to develop further as our knowledge of the complex systems regulating pancreatic function expands, eventually leading to more specialized and efficient treatments for exocrine pancreatic insufficiency.